Unhealthy healthy to healthy in six months
By
Jörgen Westin

Contents

Introduction

I was almost 46, and over the last two and a half years I had worked out at the gym twice per week with a PT. I ate good amount of salad to my meals and fruits and berries and very little sugar. Still, during my time I had worked out my weight increased five kilos and most of it was fat. I felt that I needed to change approach and test something new. This is the book of ups and downs, with what I tested and the results to where I am in August 2018. It will be workouts, food, thoughts and photos from everything during these six months.

Note: schedules are what was alright for me, but at least give you a hint on the mix between ingredients and what not to eat at all. If you have any injuries or illness, consult a doctor before you change anything from your current lifestyle.

How to make a first step to change

Already some years ago I started to go to gym and having a PT. At that point it was because of a problem with one knee. After a year with that workout my knee problem was fixed and my focus changed to be more focused on the look and thought that to achieve that a lot of the focus at the gym should be to always get stronger and be able to handle higher weights. The PT continued his schedule and yes, I got stronger and soon I could handle 140kg in deadlift. But what also happened was that my own weight increased and most of the increase was fat even though I had not eaten a lot of candy and sugar for a long time.

In the beginning of 2018 I thought that I needed to test something new. I started to wonder how? It is not easy to understand what to do yourself so help from someone is good to get. Would I get new ideas etc from my PT or would the best be to find someone else?

I decided that to really get new ideas after about two and a half year with my current PT it was time to get ideas from someone else. At the time, I thought about this I saw an ad at Facebook regarding a six months' project. It sounded to be exactly what I needed at that time.

Food

At the time, I decided to change my food intake look about this:
- Breakfast at about 06:30 on weekdays and at about 09:00 on weekends

About 3dl yoghurt with 0.5dl jam and 1dl muesli. Two bread slices with butter and cheese
- Snack after about 3 hours. Could be a banana or 2dl quark
- Lunch at about 11:45 on weekdays and at about 13:30 on weekends

A full meal where a third might be meat, a third vegetables and a third potato/pasta/rise
- Snack after about two hours. Could be a banana or 2dl quark
- Dinner at about 18:00

A full meal like the lunch. Meat about 250g before cooking.
- If hungry in the evening at about 20:00 to 21:00 a snack which could be quark, yoghurt or often two slices of bread

I have learned that three meals with snacks in between was good for someone working out so I ate like that. Also some sauce to meat and the yoghurt was standard with 3% fat etc. I was often hungry in the evenings so the snack at that time was more like a rule.

Workout

I worked out two times per week at the gym, always with a PT. Often mostly focusing on lower or upper body, but with one or two other workouts and some pulse training. No day was like previous days, so workouts looped around in a way where one type of workout could be weeks from the last time. On top of the gym workouts I like to walk and explore so often walking at least 20km per week.

First meeting February 6

I did not know what to expect when I went to the first meeting for this project. I knew it was a meeting for the trainer to understand my goals and my status, and for me to get a schedule for food and workouts as well as being measured the first time.

It all started with discussions regarding my goals. The goals I mentioned were a bit different to most I think. I did not have a goal on losing weight nor lift X kilos etc. My goals were a look (I was showing a picture of a man I thought looked very good) and a better health.

Then it was time for measuring. The weight I knew well, and this day it ended up at 80kg. The other measurements I have always thought be hard to do correct yourself, but here is what it was at the first meeting:

Shoulders	>	**114cm**
Chest	>	**94cm**
Waist	>	**91cm**
Belly button	>	**93.5cm**
Hip	>	**93cm**
Thigh	>	**53cm**
Upper arm	>	**30cm**

Also at every meeting with the trainer it would be a body fat calculation, something I have never done before. At this first measurement, this where the figures:

Collarbone	>	**8mm**
Stomach	>	**33.8mm**
Thigh	>	**12.1mm**
Triceps	>	**11.2mm**
Shoulder blade	>	**15.2mm**
Hip	>	**24.3mm**
Ribs	>	**21mm**
Bodyfat	>	**20.20%**

The trainer tried to be nice and said that the figures were not flattering and a lot should be different.

The trainer then started to talk about food and if I ever had thought about testing the 16/8 diet where you eat all meals for a day during 8 hours, and no calories on the other 16 hours. He gave me links to info about this method for example links to scientists which have also been discover in big science magazines as well as partly being involved in science for resulting in a Nobel prize. After I have read it I said to the trainer that I would like to test it.

So the trainer put together a schedule for me, for food and workouts, to get the results I wanted within six months. Note: All schedules changing food radically with avoiding or adding something should be after suggestion from a person with education in nutrition, especially if you have some illness, injury or diabetes etc.

Starting schedules I got from the trainer below in Food and Workout.

Food

The first schedule for the 16/8 diet had a focus on losing fat without losing muscles.

Meal 1 and 3

Protein	Example in schedule was 200g cooked/grilled/stir-fried meat (note it is cooked weight, not as in many other diets the raw weight)
Carbohydrate	About 1 dl rise or pasta, or 1.5dl potatoes
Fat	2 tablespoons of low fat dressing/quark
Salad	Up to 300g

Meal 2

Protein	Example 200g low fat quark
Carbohydrate	About 1dl grains
Fat	Example 1 egg

The trainer explained that the mix and amounts will match almost what athletes use when they are in the period to get shredded.

The trainer said: "You will the first weeks be very hungry at times when you should not eat, then drink a cup of coffee or water (or sugar free soda)."

A more complete list I got (Note: schedule is what was alright for me, but at least give you a hint on the mix between ingredients and what not to eat at all) where I should pick one from each section

Meal 1 and 3

Protein	200g of cooked/grilled/stir-fried meat
	From cow, pig, bird, fish, moose/deer, shell fish or soya/qourn/tofu
Carbohydrate	170g potatoes or sweet potatoes
	90g rise or quinoa or bulgur
	80g pasta or seeds (wheat and similar)
	110g potatoes or sweet potatoes in oven
	120g beans
	200g root vegetables
	500g wok vegetables
Fat	1 egg
	Half avocado
	15g nuts
	20g pesto
	30g butter (40%)
	35g cheese (17%)
	40g mozzarella or feta (20%)
	50g cheese (10%) or olives or crème fraiche (15%)
	75g Turkish yoghurt
	1dl coconut milk light
	1 tablespoon oil
Salad	Up to 300g (not corn) with max 1-2 tablespoon low fat dressing/sauce

Meal 2

Protein	200g quark
	200g cottage cheese
	70g low fat cheese
	1 portion protein powder
Carbohydrates	1dl grains or müsli
	1 slice of dark bread
	1 banana
	200g wild berries
	1 mango
	2 oranges
Fat	1 egg
	1 table spoon peanut butter
	15g seeds
	30g butter max 40% fat
	50g soft cheese max 15% fat

Workout

The workout schedule I got was based upon a few exercises for upper and lower body. We discussed how I usually like to split workouts during a week and we came up with a mix of two days with upper body and two days with lower body per week, and never two upper or two lower after each other. On top of that to start burn some more fat I should either take a pulse increasing walk for an hour per day, or something similar.

The suggested set up in the gym was to do 4 sets on each exercise, with decreasing number of reps per set and increasing the weight for each set. Suggested number of reps were 12, 10, 8 and 6 for the four sets. What weight to use I needed to test and found out. The weight should be exactly the weight I managed for the set. All exercises should be performed with good technique and slowly, or at least slowly in one direction (for example leg press can be a fast push out, and then slowly going back). I got the instruction that the technique and the speed (=slow) were very important to get a good increase in muscle mass and do it without injure myself.

All workouts at the gym were "machine free", just weights etc. Here is the list of workouts:

Upper body
Chins
Dumbell press
Dumbell row
Military press
Dumbell flyes
Dumbell side lifts
Something for biceps and triceps
Lower body
Barbell squats
Barbell deadlifts
Lunges
Leg press
Something for abs: sit ups, leg raises, plank....

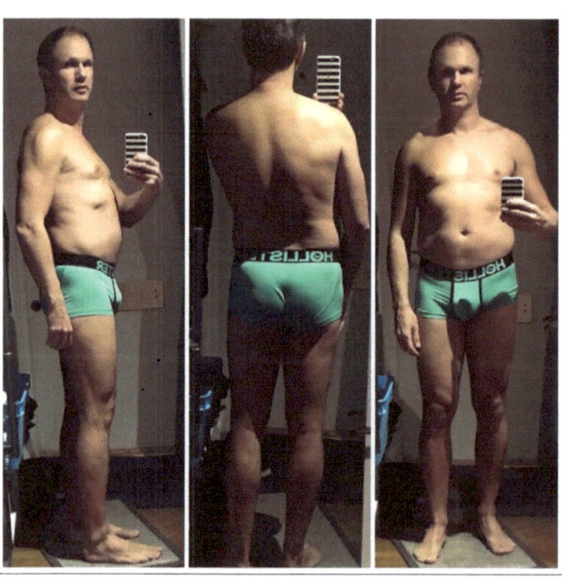

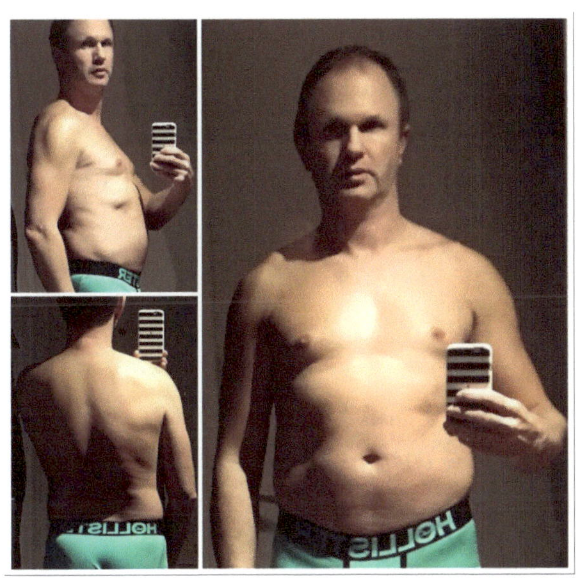

First week

First week was a bit challenging for several reasons. First to adjust and understand how to eat. Weighing the food and try to learn how it looks on a plate = learn the size of protein, carbo hydrates and fat I should have to avoid weighing everything. Also the food was a bit challenging because I have learned from parents that breakfast is the most important meal of the day, and now I am avoiding breakfast completely. I got hungry a lot a few days on times when I should not eat anything, so there was a need for coffee, water or "zero" sugar soda. But it was easier than I expected anyway to make the change partly I think because I am single and a bit stubborn, so if I decide something I will do it and as a single I do not need to adjust to anyone else's need.

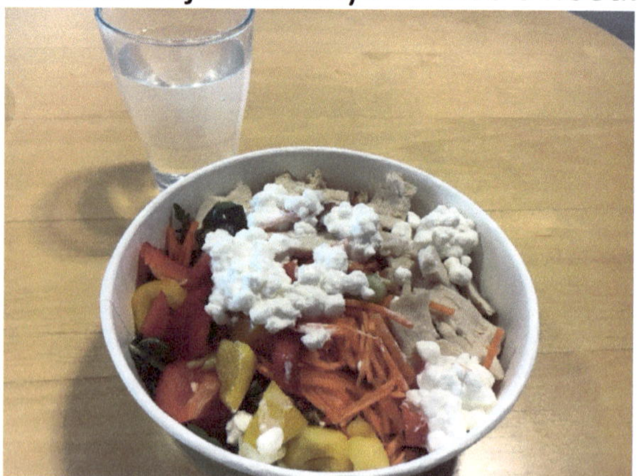

Workout

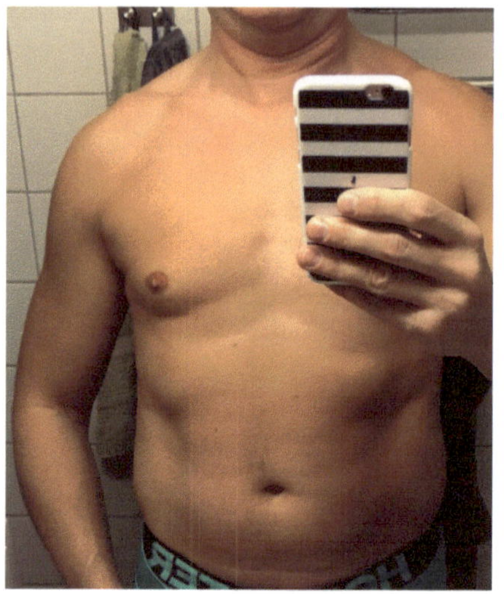

I really tried to follow the workout schedule directly for at least two days per week for the gym, and about 4-5 days per week regarding the walk. I quickly found out that the way to get so much walking done I need to use the belt in the gym and walk there for an hour. Often, I did it in the morning and even though I now did not eat any breakfast it felt like I had the energy. The gym workouts the two days I did not follow the schedule was a bit more varied with different exercises. The two days I followed the schedule I first walked an hour and then did the exercises, so I spent about two hours at the gym. Still felt a lot of energy. Did not add anything else then some BCAA to drink.

First temptation, work related trip to Spain

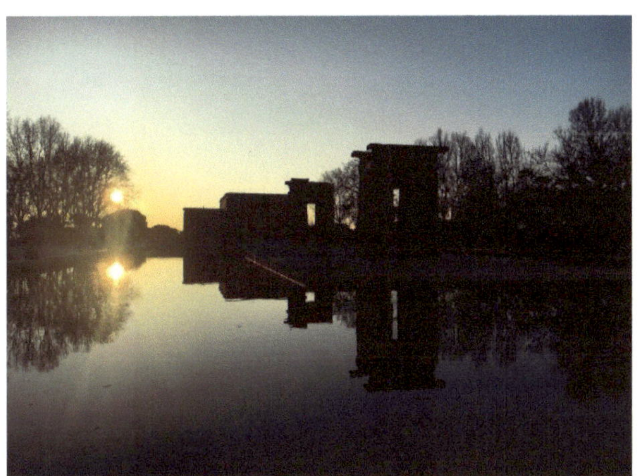

Soon after I have started with this six months' project there was a work trip to Madrid. Work trips are generally not good for the health, it is long days with unhealthy food and perhaps some party in the evening. So this was really a temptation. I had got a rather good feeling for how 200g meat looks like etc so the way I handled the food at the trip was that I did not avoid every dessert or avoid every treat, but if I took something which were not in the schedule I compensated by reducing carbo hydrates etc. The trip was just four days so even if I maybe would not manage to do a good job it would not damage everything.

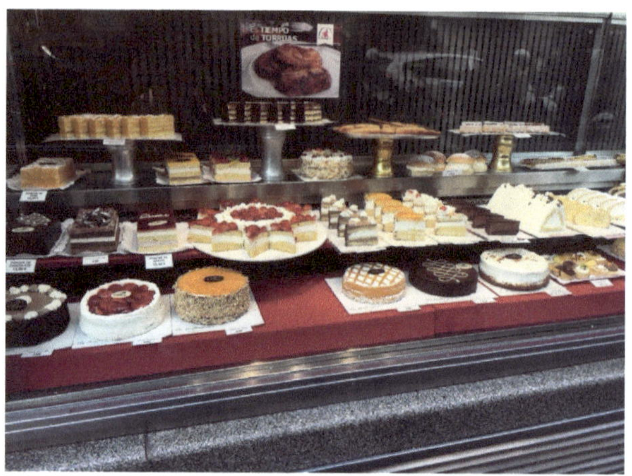

So how did I do? Because I have changed to the 16/8 food schedule it worked well anyway, I came home weighing less despite a not perfect food intake and despite the lack of workouts.

The first month

The first month was tough, I had never in my life done so much walking and workouts. I saw on the scale that almost every day I lost about 200g weight. Some days I could not follow the schedule completely because I either had not the time or strength to completely follow it. So I already from the start thought about what to make less of if I cannot do everything. Also there was sometimes a queue in the gym for some spaces to use dumbbells on a bench so I started for myself to wonder what I either could do less of or exchange to something else if I needed, and still do exercises for the right muscles. So here is what I found out I could change some times:

Chins	> **Less, skip or Lats machine**
Dumbbell press	> **Chest press machine**
Dumbbell flyes	> **Flyes machine**

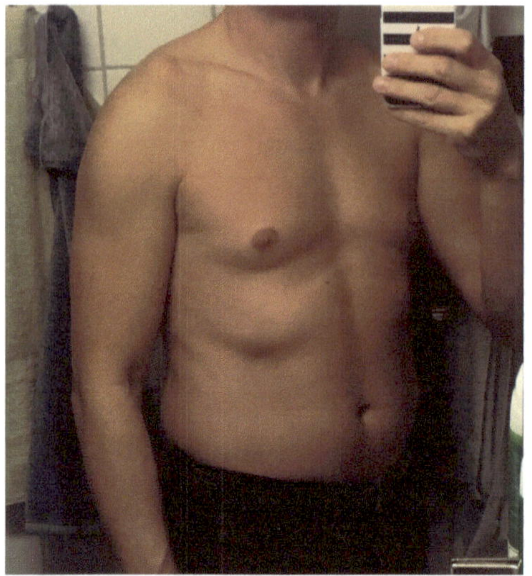

For the biceps and triceps, I often added curls in machines.

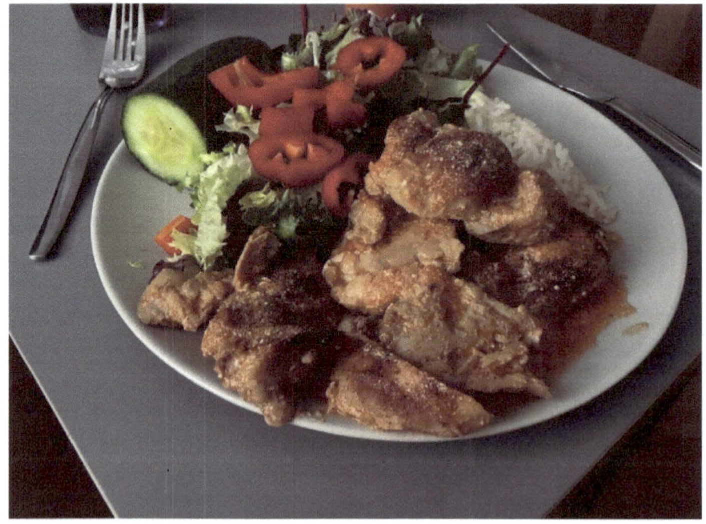

The food went very well during this month and I was really keeping carbohydrates and fat to a minimum.

First results

When it was time for getting the first results I was a bit nervous, had I done a good job or not. I turned up at the gym and we started the measurements.

		Now	Start
Shoulders	>	**113.5cm**	114cm
Chest	>	**93cm**	94cm
Waist	>	**78cm**	91cm
Belly button	>	**82cm**	93.5cm
Hip	>	**92cm**	93cm
Thigh	>	**52cm**	53cm
Upper arm	>	**30.5cm**	30cm

Collarbone	>	**5.8mm**	8mm
Stomach	>	**22.1mm**	33.8mm
Thigh	>	**9.3mm**	12.1mm
Triceps	>	**7.4mm**	11.2mm
Shoulder blade	>	**11.4mm**	15.2mm
Hip	>	**17.2mm**	24.3mm
Ribs	>	**14.7mm**	21mm
Bodyfat	>	**14.70%**	20.20%

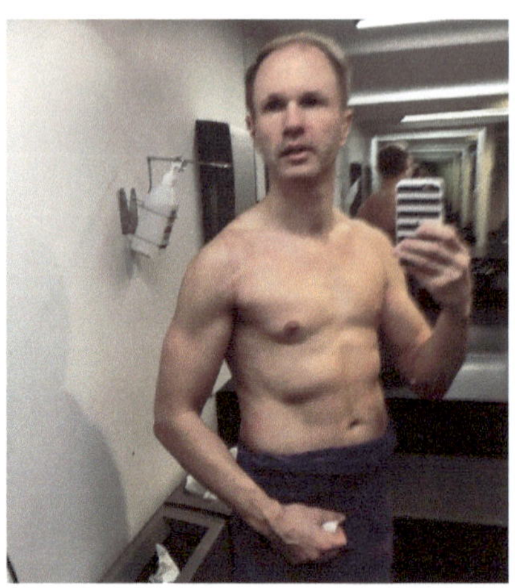

I was surprised about the results, better than I expected. The weight had dropped from 80kg to 74kg. So considering that drop, and the decreased waist and bodyfat, it was not any surprise for the trainer that some parts of the body where muscles should be gained had decreased a bit.

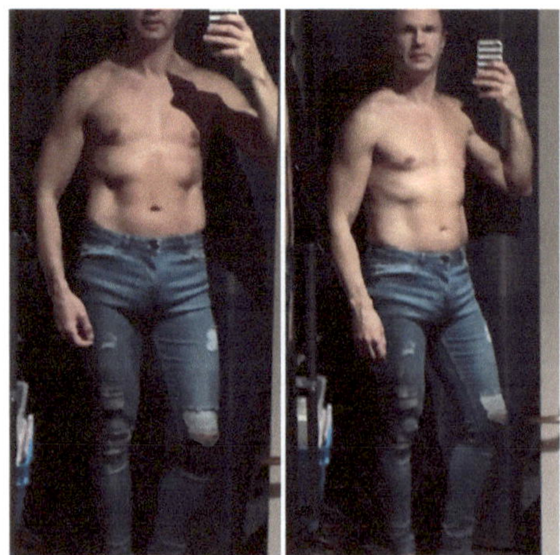

Because the weight had dropped 6kg and the bodyfat so much in just a month the food scheduled was changed a bit. The protein part for meal 1 and two increased from 200g to 300g. The trainer thought everything dropped a bit too fast.

No big changes in the workout schedule.

Second temptation, holiday to Gran Canaria

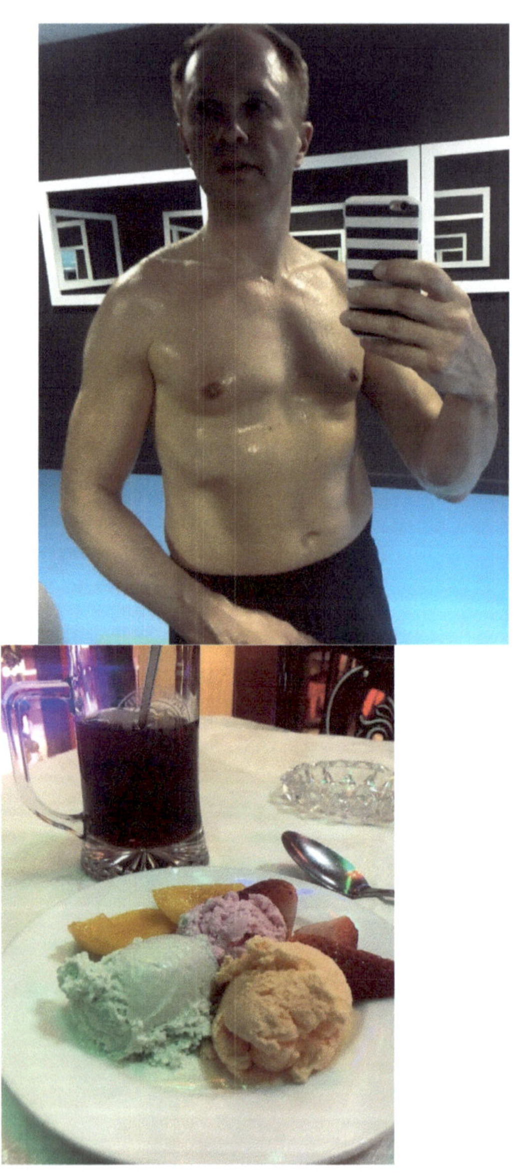

Not long after the measurements I was going on a trip to Gran Canaria with sun, relaxing and party. A real temptation. I was travelling alone and had chosen a hotel with a gym and where you could cook your own food in the room. I could still skip breakfast, cook my own food at lunch and eat dinner out in the evenings. So at least it was not totally unhealthy, but too much fat, some drinks and too much carbohydrates. To compensate I was at the gym every morning even though it was really hot. Thanks to the heat and 45 minutes walking I still lost weight and fat. Not perfect with food and training but I learned that it is possible to still enjoy life and keep on towards my goal.

Second month

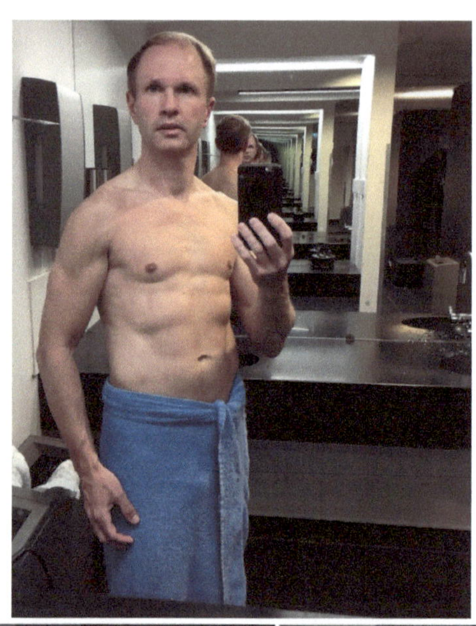

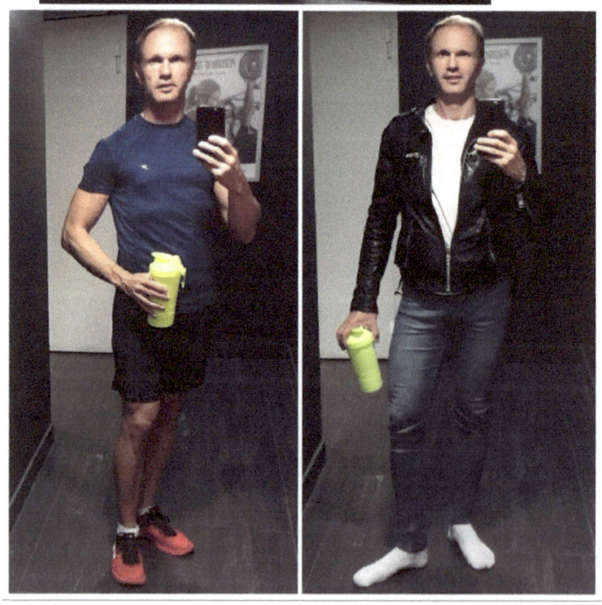

When I came home from that trip to Gran Canaria I was full of energy. I saw that it was possible to do nice things and still in the end be healthy. I started to work out even more so some weeks I was at the gym for 5 to 6 days per week. Often 3-4 days with upper body and 1-2 days with lower body. I had found out that lower body needed more recovery time and that some parts on the upper body grew to slowly. I started to almost avoid any extra walking after a suggestion from the trainer via email, because he thought that I do not need to drop fat or weight any faster.

Second results

In May it was time for new results. I was not sure at all about the status before the meeting. I think it is very hard to use a tape and measure at the right spots on the body yourself. If I try twice the results can differ 5cm. So I hoped that it would be good, because when I looked in the mirror it looked good.

		Now	Start
Shoulders	>	**113cm**	114cm
Chest	>	**92cm**	94cm
Waist	>	**78cm**	91cm
Belly button	>	**78cm**	93.5cm
Hip	>	**91cm**	93cm
Thigh	>	**51cm**	53cm
Upper arm	>	**31cm**	30cm

Collarbone	>	**4.4mm**	8mm
Stomach	>	**12.3mm**	33.8mm
Thigh	>	**8mm**	12.1mm
Triceps	>	**6.2mm**	11.2mm
Shoulder blade	>	**9mm**	15.2mm
Hip	>	**9.2mm**	24.3mm
Ribs	>	**8.9mm**	21mm
Bodyfat	>	**10.10%**	20.20%

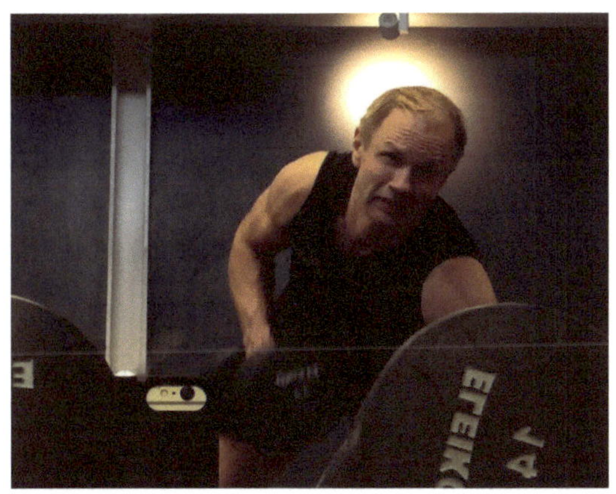

It was amazing results. In about 2.5 months the bodyfat had decreased to half of what I started with and the weight was now 72.1kg, 7.9kg less than what I started with. The trainer said that I should stop any extra walks, and for the food it was changed so that I should double meal 2. More than that he did not think was possible to eat.

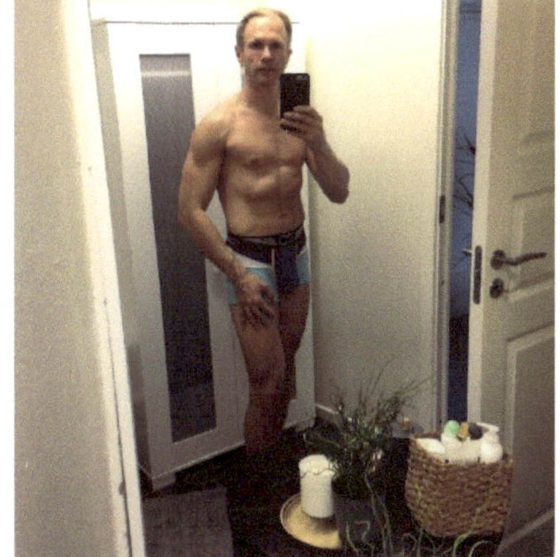

When the trainer saw the results and that some body parts decreased which we wanted to increase he said that I should try adding a PWO drink before my workouts, to get the extra energy for the muscles to do their very best during the workouts. He also said that if I had it hard some times to eat all what I should, then I should add some protein powder.

That was all the changes he recommended.

Change in approach

After that meeting with the trainer I started to experiment a bit more myself. I added more different types of exercises to pick from, I started to do more exercises per day and I started to test if 12, 10, 8 and 6 reps were the best for me. I was more confident myself now on what was needed so I thought that tests of new things never could damage the way to my goal.

I started to see that it felt like 10, 8, 6,4 reps often gave me more and could push me to really use higher and higher weights in the gym.

I changed so that no day had the same order of the exercises, even if it was the same exercises I used.

I experimented by doing a weekly schedule repeating this:

Upper   Lower   Upper   Rest

I soon had a list of about 20 exercises for upper body (mostly machines at that point) and about 15 exercises for lower body. Usually I took 6-9 exercises from the list to execute on a workout day.

The original schedule talked about at least 1 minute rest between sets, I usually now had more than that, often 2-3 minutes. Instead pushing to very high weights and doing the exercises slowly, which is tough and will get you into an intense breathing.

My list of exercises:

Upper body
Abs machine
Bench press
Bench press incline
Biceps curl machine
Biceps curl standing cables
Chest press machine
Chest press incline machine
Chins
Chins narrow
Dumbbell flyes
Dumbbell press
Dumbbell press incline
Dumbbell row
Dumbbell side lift
Flyes machine
Lats machine, bending in
Lats machine, straight
Low row machine
Military press
Push ups
Raised push ups
Shoulder press machine
Shoulder raise machine
Triceps curl machine
Z bar curl
Lower body
Abductor machine
Adductor machine
Barbell squat
Calves machine
Deadlift
Leg curl laying down machine
Leg curl sitting machine
Leg extension machine
Leg press, push body
Leg press, push legs
Lunges
Plank
Sumo deadlift

Third temptation, holiday to Gran Canaria

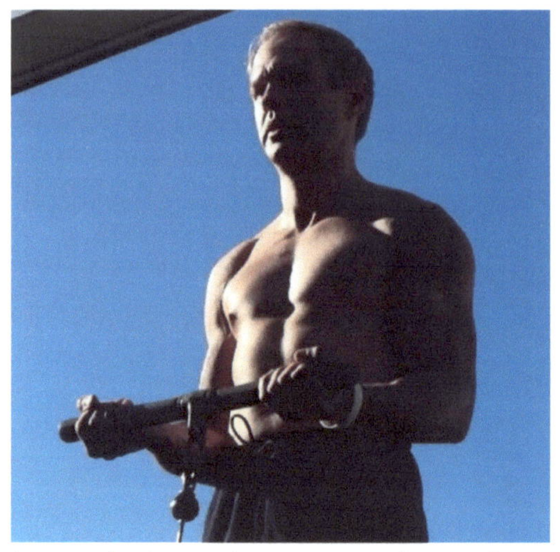

In early June I went to Gran Canaria again. I booked a hotel which called itself "...wellness" and they talked about their outdoor gym, so I thought it would be perfect. Not much of a gym but at least I tested it the first day, instead I went to a real gym outdoor just a few hundred metres away and went to that gym every morning before doing something else. Really hot even in the mornings but it went really well in that gym. I could almost do everything like at home and I still followed the diet and did not eat breakfast. So in total I actually lost weight and felt stronger when I checked at home directly after the trip.

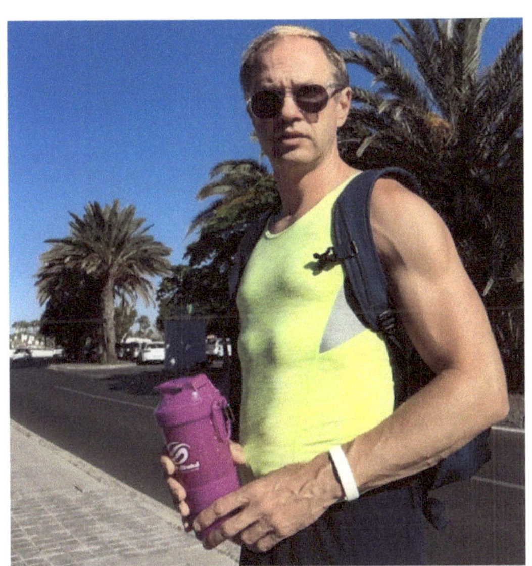

Did I cheat at the trip, regarding food – yes. I did not cheat regarding breakfast, but lunch and dinner was not perfect. It was sometimes not only 8 hours of eating/drinking time, it could be even 12. It was too much desserts and some alcohol almost every day.

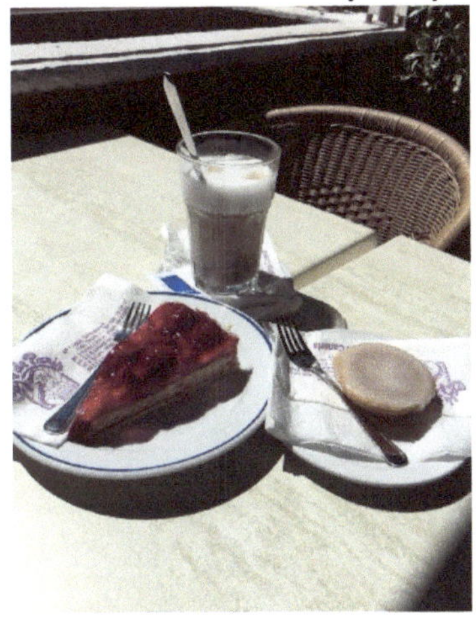

So did it affect something to cheat like this? Yes, but not on body weight. I felt however when I was back home that the body felt heavier for a couple of weeks. But you need to have these types of trips sometimes as well, you just need to stop cheating after the trip and to be aware of how you cheated – not lie to yourself.

Summer heat slow down results

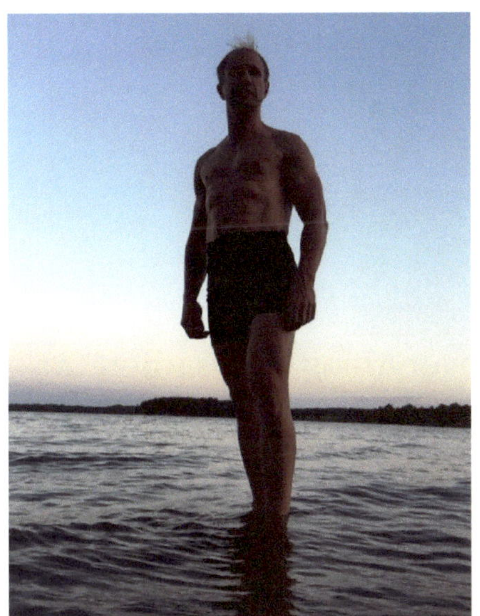

When I was back home the real heat started in Sweden this summer. So long period with about 20 degrees in the nights and 28 in the day shadow is very rare. I tested to do workouts in other times, tried to have double rest periods between sets etc. It helped a bit but week after week with that heat really affected the body. It was hard to eat the correct amount of food as well, so it was often some protein powder added to daily food intake.

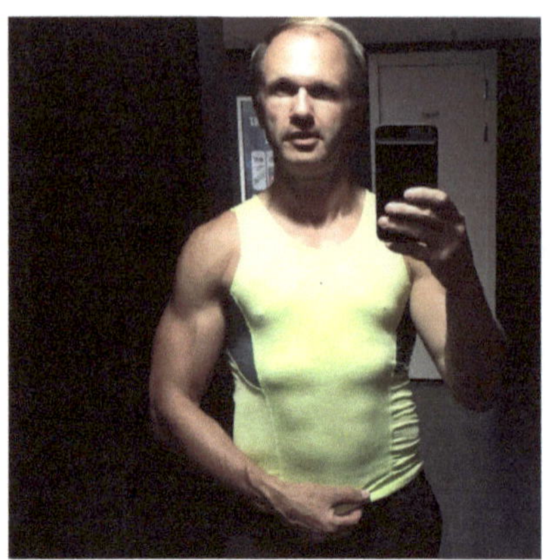

Despite that I felt everything was harder, for almost six weeks I almost every time at the gym set a record in something. It went well a very long time. But then, in the middle of the summer heat I started to feel a hunger for sweet things. Something I had not felt for many years. I started to add some cakes, it was a lot of ice creams in the heat etc. I started to notice that my body changed and was afraid it was due to this with the desserts etc. My weight was 76kg, about 4kg heavier than the last time I was away and measured everything. I really started to be scared that I had ruined my good results. I started to decrease the sugar intake again and was soon at 74.5kg. But at that weight it seemed to stop, and I thought that I had a problem and my "six pack" was not as visible anymore either.

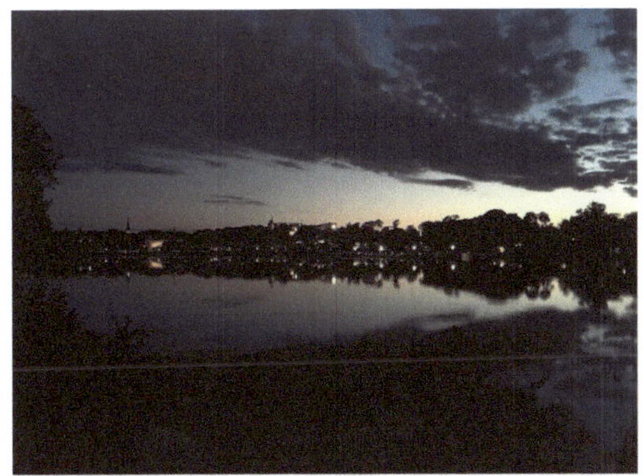

    Except going back to low sugar food I was more careful again with the intake of carbohydrates.

Preparing for August results

I did continue trying get back in shape as I thought. But on the other hand, when I took some pictures I thought I looked much more muscled but maybe not with very defined muscles. So what was the truth? The preparation was changed a bit. I started to do more focused workouts, focusing just on a few things I thought needed workouts the most: the chest, shoulders and back. A lot of the focus on the chest because I thought that if I cannot make my waist thinner in an easy way, make the chest bigger and the V-shape will be there. No matter what I did, the weight was between 74-75kg all the time.

Half year summary

So came the moment of truth. Time for another measurement after the six months had passed. Did I achieve my goals? How was the status? What next?

The weight was the first thing, 74.9kg. Both me and the trainer started to think, has it been some bad summer months? Then the rest of the measurements:

		Now	Start
Shoulders	>	115.5cm	114cm
Chest	>	94cm	94cm
Waist	>	79.5cm	91cm
Belly button	>	80.5cm	93.5cm
Hip	>	93cm	93cm
Thigh	>	52.5cm	53cm
Upper arm	>	32.5cm	30cm

		Now	Start
Collarbone	>	4.8mm	8mm
Stomach	>	12.7mm	33.8mm
Thigh	>	8.4mm	12.1mm
Triceps	>	6.6mm	11.2mm
Shoulder blade	>	10.1mm	15.2mm
Hip	>	9.6mm	24.3mm
Ribs	>	9.4mm	21mm
Bodyfat	>	10.70%	20.20%

We both were surprised. It was better than we both thought it would be. Increasing centimetres in some important areas, keeping other parts in an ok state and having the bodyfat in a very good place. The trainer has said earlier that if the bodyfat went from 10.1% as in May to just over 12% it would still be good, and now it still was under 11% and had increased some sizes and increased weight with 2.8kg. That combined means that I had increased muscle mass with over 2kg….

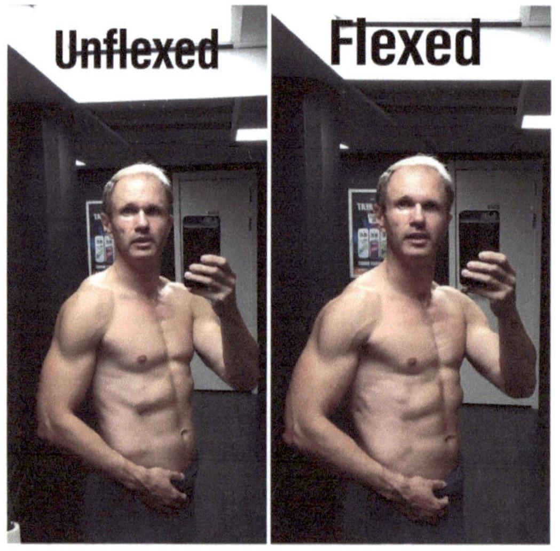

Was I achieving my goals during these 6 months? Yes, the goal with better health and a goal for the look I achieved already after half the time. I had exceeded the goals.

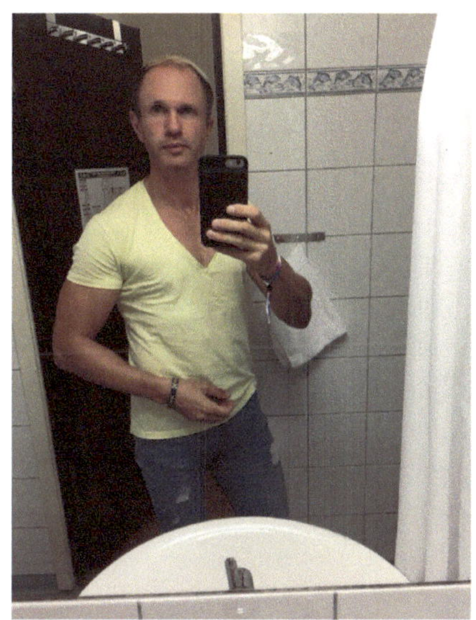

What did the trainer think? He thought that I had done something rather unusual – down to about 10% body fat (half from start) and 2+ kg muscles in six months. For many that takes at least 18 months. He just said that "keep on going like this, I have no more advise for the moment. Expect 1 to 2 kilos increased muscle mass per year".

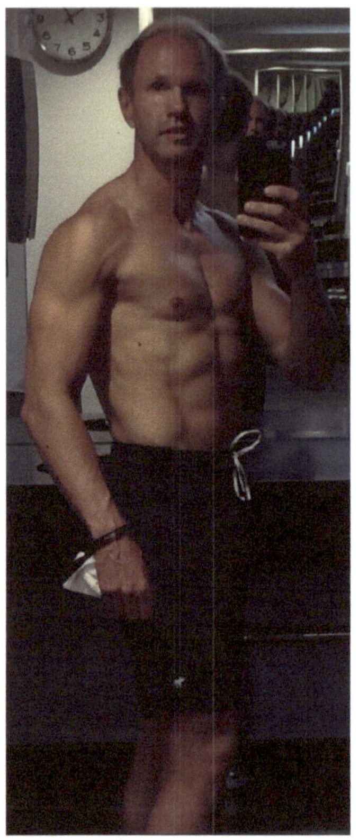

Was I using some other supplements or steroids etc to achieve this? No, I have only used BCAA with glutamine around my workouts, PWO before the workouts for some extra energy and when I have not been able to eat enough protein some protein power shakes. Nothing else.

How it will continue

So how will this continue? Of course, I need to have some goals, everyone needs that to achieve something. The goals should be realistic. I am thinking of what my goals will be for the next half year ending in February (=total one year from start). My short-term goal is to work on the V-shape and the six pack. No need for a goal on achieving X kg in some workouts. For me it is not a goal to be strong.

Food

From all I have learned during the six months I now know how it is possible to temporarily cheat and still reach the goals afterwards. I also know how to get more shredded to a summer for example, by going back to the food schedule I started with, and eat like that maybe 2 months before the summer. I also know that the food schedule I have now is really working for me and I can keep using it.

Workouts

I do not plan to change much in the workouts. I might adjust/add to the list of exercises if I found something new but I have all basics there.

The only thing I think is that I will more often to more focused workouts, with maybe more sets and less reps with really heavy weights, to see what that will give. But about 4 days per week, with about 6 exercises per day is what I see will be the right quantity right now.

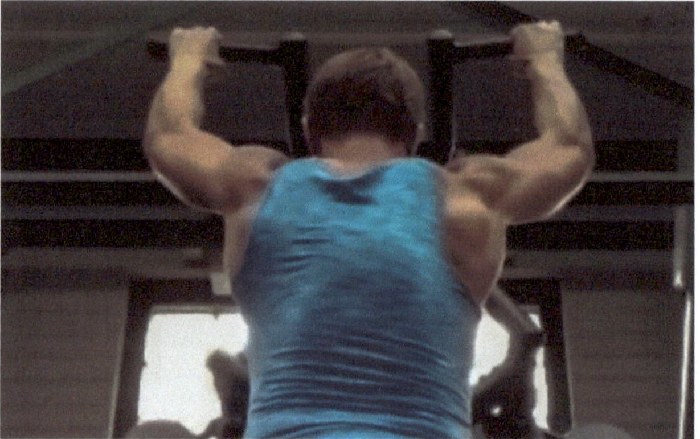

The standard workouts will most likely be:

Upper body
Abs machine
Biceps curl machine
Chest press machine
Dumbbell press incline
Dumbbell side lift
Flyes machine
Lats machine, bending in
Shoulder press machine
Triceps curl machine
Lower body
Barbell squat
Calves machine
Deadlift or sumo dedlift
Leg curl sitting machine
Leg extension machine
Leg press, puch legs

Supplements

As I said I have not used much. Is there something I like to add? Not necessary, if it would be something it might be something to "repair/build muscles" after workout and maybe some vitamins/minerals.

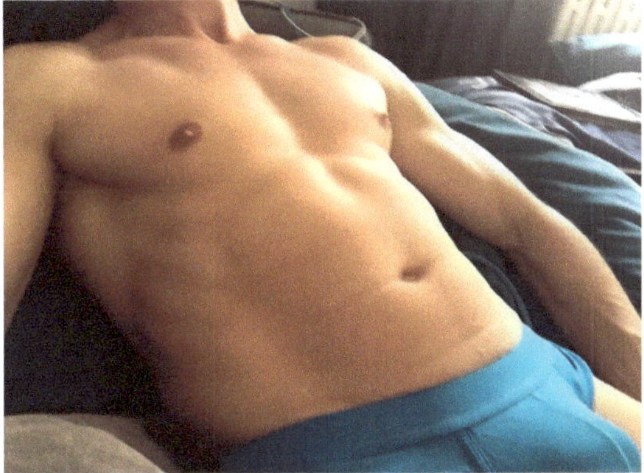

But in general I think that the best is to not add so much, focusing just on good food and the correct training.

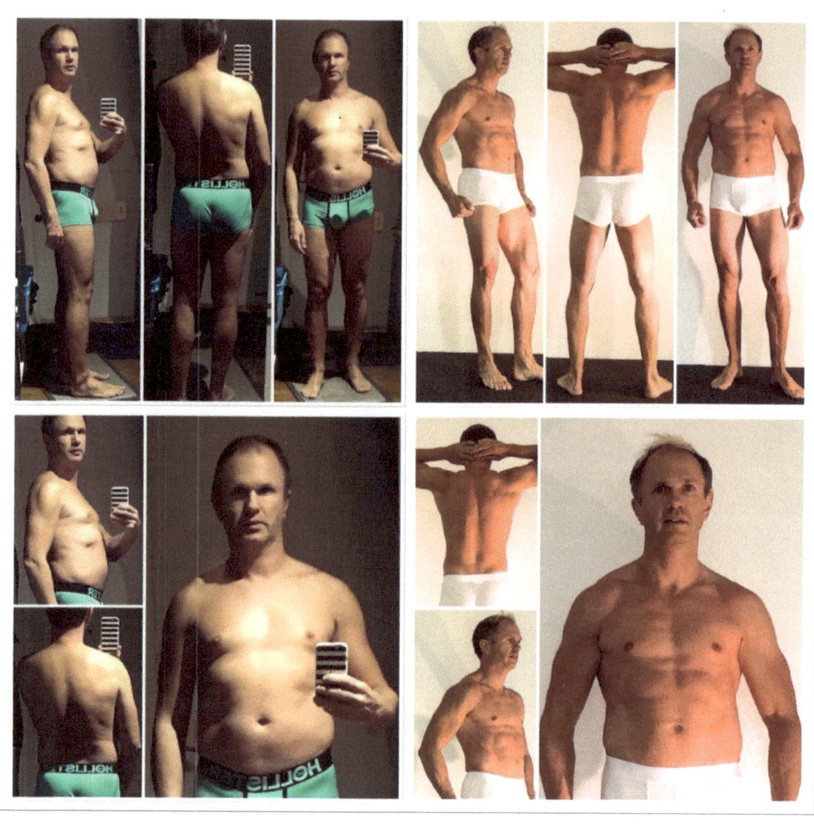

Workout schedule made after 6 months

After the six months, below is the main general workout schedule I will use. My body needs more rest between each lower body workout so it will be more upper vs lower body in the schedule.

If the 7th day is not a resting day, the week after should start with a resting day instead and the rest of the days in schedule moved forward (Day 1 becomes Day 2, Day 2 becomes Day 3 etc).

	Day 1 Upper body	Day 2 Lower body	Day 3 Upper body	Day 4 Rest	Day 5 Upper body	Day 6 Rest	Day 7 Rest or Combo upper/lower
1	Chest press incline machine	Deadlift or Sumo deadlift	Dumbbell press incline		Chest press incline machine		Pushups
2	Flyes machine	Leg press, push legs	Dumbbell row		Dumbbell press incline		Abs machine
3	Lats machine, bending in	Calves machine	Dumbbell press		Dumbbell press		Leg press, push legs
4	Abs machine	Leg curl sitting machine	Shoulder raise machine		Flyes machine		Leg extension machine
5	Biceps curl machine	Leg extension machine	Biceps curl machine		Shoulder raise machine		
6	Triceps curl machine	Abs machine	Triceps curl machine		Abs machine		
7	Add 1 from list below	Add 1 from list below	Abs machine		Add 1 from list below		
8			Add 1 from list below				
	4 sets:	4 sets:	4 sets:		4 sets:		4 sets:
	12x60%	12x60%	10x70%		10x70%		10x70%
	10x70%	10x70%	10x80%		10x80%		10x80%
	8x80%	8x80%	8x90%		8x90%		8x90%
	6x90-110%	6x90-110%	6x90-110%		6x90-110%		6x90-110%

Note: Percentage is from your previous max. All reps and weights should be adjusted for how it feels for the day.
The goal is that set 3 and 4 should be exactly what you can manage for that day.

Abs machine
Bench press
Bench press incline
Biceps curl machine
Biceps curl standing cables
Chest press machine
Chest press incline machine
Chins
Chins narrow
Dumbbell flyes
Dumbbell press
Dumbbell press incline
Dumbbell row
Dumbbell side lift
Flyes machine
Lats machine, bending in
Lats machine, straight
Low row machine
Military press
Push ups
Raised push ups
Shoulder press machine
Shoulder raise machine
Triceps curl machine
Z bar curl
Lower body
Abductor machine
Adductor machine
Barbell squat
Calves machine
Deadlift
Leg curl laying down machine
Leg curl sitting machine
Leg extension machine
Leg press, push body
Leg press, push legs
Lunges
Plank
Sumo deadlift

www.ingramcontent.com/pod-product-compliance
Lightning Source LLC
Chambersburg PA
CBHW040214240726
48664CB00019B/1398